Foreword

Although the U.S. is one of the wealthiest nations in the world, we are far from being the healthiest, and consistently lag behind other developed nations in life expectancy and other population health measures. These disparities prevail despite the fact that the U.S. spends more dollars per capita than any other nation on healthcare delivery. However, simply fixing the U.S. healthcare delivery system (though sorely needed) or putting additional resources into precision medicine initiatives (though useful for subsets of patients), will likely fall short of improving the overall health of the U.S. population. This is because the country is suffering primarily from chronic medical conditions, such as heart disease, obesity, and type 2 diabetes. These non-communicable diseases are largely the result of individual behaviors and lifestyle choices made in the context of a low physical activity, high calorie environment. In fact, a recent JAMA study concludes that "In many cases, the best investments for improving population health would likely be public health programs and multispectral action to address risks such as physical inactivity, diet, ambient particulate pollution, and alcohol and tobacco consumption."

In this publication, Dr. Michael Joyner and colleagues reach similar conclusions and provide a roadmap to address lifestyle factors that are best for healthspan (the period of life free of chronic diseases). These lifestyle factors can help ensure the highest quality of health for the longest period of life. Although the publication addresses the three primary causes of non-communicable chronic diseases – tobacco use, poor diet, and lack of proper physical activity, particular emphasis is placed on addressing physical inactivity. Numerous studies suggest that physical activity can compensate for other poor behaviors, yet about 50% of children and greater than 90% of adults and seniors do not meet the daily U.S. guidelines for physical activity. This lack of physical activity, combined with other lifestyle factors, has placed the U.S. on a difficult roadmap. The lack of physical activity route is unsustainable and characterized by high healthcare costs with a lower level of health for the population. Something must be done to get the county back on track and improve the overall health of our population, as well as the fiscal state of the nation. The roadmap presented by Joyner and colleagues in this publication does just that. It is not only viable, but actionable today. Healthcare professionals, policy-makers, and concerned citizens should pay heed to their point of view.

Frank Booth, PhD

Professor of Biomedical Sciences, University of Missouri

Founder of Researchers Against Inactivity Related Diseases (RID)

July 2015

Preface

A Roadmap to Better Health is a book of ideas and data presented in chart format about what can be done to improve the health of the population of the United States and by extension many other countries that literally "suffer" from the effects of a low physical activity, high calorie world. It emerged from a long running and ongoing e-mail exchange among the authors that began in 2012. Although the initial focus of our conversation had something to do with the quality, coverage, and costs of the so-called health care system in the U.S., it soon became clear that many of these issues were inseparable from the root causes of most chronic non-communicable diseases, root causes which are largely behavioral and environmental. Thus we began to search for strategies that could promote healthy behaviors in individuals, communities, and the society as a whole.

To support our emerging ideas we looked to the scientific literature and other sources that could help us highlight "what might be done" and "what has been shown to work". In this context, the fundamental idea underpinning our book is that increases in most people's physical activity level is the key to both better individual and population health. To achieve this goal, we propose a three-pronged approach of environmental, economic, and educational "nudges", highlighting the idea that broad based action is required at levels ranging from the personal all the way to public policy.

We hope that *A Roadmap to Better Health* is useful to a wide audience but especially to healthcare professionals and policy makers. More importantly, we hope that it stimulates discussion on common sense and low costs steps that can be used to improve the health of individual Americans and also help reduce health care costs to society as a whole.

Michael J. Joyner, MD
Professor of Anesthesiology, Mayo Clinic

July 2015

Note: This work reflects the perspectives of the individual authors and does not necessarily represent the opinions of their respective institutions - Arizona State University and Mayo Clinic.

Table of contents

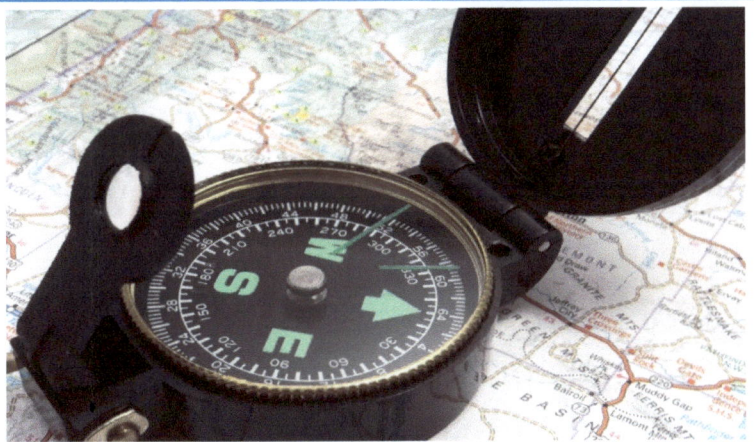

A ROADMAP TO BETTER HEALTH

July 2015

Outline

1. Executive summary
2. The U.S. needs better health but healthcare delivery is not the answer
3. What has worked
4. Where to start

Our premise and objectives

- The U.S. needs:
  - A healthy population
  - A high-value healthcare delivery system
- However, a healthy population and high-value healthcare delivery are not the same
- Here we focus primarily on the main determinants of **health** to help U.S. citizens and leaders establish a roadmap to a healthier population

3

First, what do we mean by *health*?

"**Health** is a state of complete physical, mental and social well-being and not merely the absence of disease or infirmity."

-World Health Organization (WHO)

Source: WHO. "WHO definition of health." http://www.who.int/about/definition/en/print.html (accessed March 16, 2015).

4

Healthcare delivery is a minor determinant of overall health; Individual behavior is key

Key determinants of the health of a population

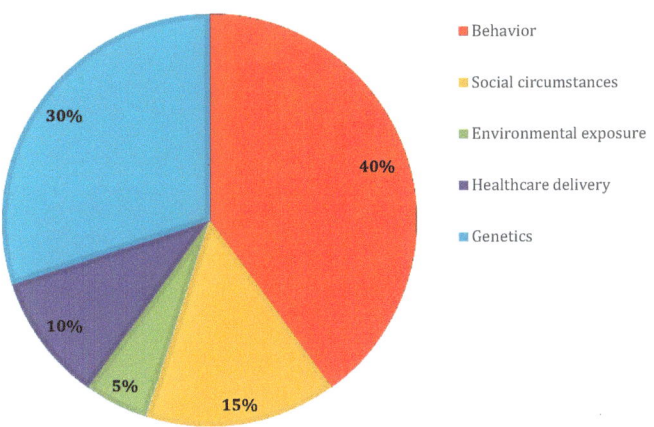

- ■ Behavior
- ■ Social circumstances
- ■ Environmental exposure
- ■ Healthcare delivery
- ■ Genetics

Source: McGinnis et al. 2002. "The case for more active policy attention to health promotion." *Health Affairs* 21(2): 78-93.

Note: Estimates of the determinants of overall health vary widely, for alternate estimates see http://www.kingsfund.org.uk/time-to-think-differently/trends/broader-determinants-health,http://www.cdc.gov/socialdeterminants/FAQ.html, or http://www.health.state.mn.us/divs/opi/gov/chsadmin/intro.html. However, all estimates generally postulate a predominant role for factors other than traditional "healthcare" or genetics.

We all know what to do to stay healthy: Follow Lester Breslow's 7 Healthy Habits!

1. Don't smoke or abuse drugs
2. Eat a balanced and healthy diet
3. Get regular exercise and control your weight
4. Do not drink a lot of alcohol
5. Take care of your teeth
6. Manage high blood pressure
7. Follow good safety practices

And yet...

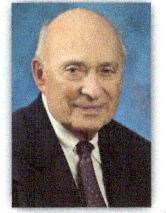

Note: Dr. Lester Breslow was a major leader in the field of public health for nearly seven decades. Among many positions held, he served as the dean of the Fielding School of Public Health at UCLA.
Source: Van Voorhees, B. 2007. "Healthy habits." http://www.nytimes.com/health/guides/specialtopic/healthy-living/overview.html (accessed December 16, 2014). Photo credit: UCLA Fielding School of Public Health.

Despite significant progress, >40 million Americans still regularly smoke cigarettes

U.S. adults who smoke cigarettes (1965-2012)
Percent

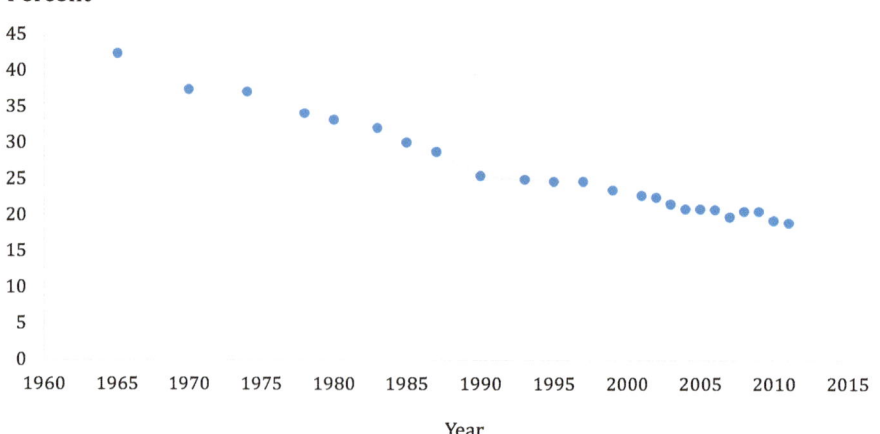

Source: CDC. 2013. "Trends in current cigarette smoking among high school students and adults, United States, 1965-2011." http://www.cdc.gov/tobacco/data_statistics/tables/trends/cig_smoking/index.htm (accessed November 12, 2014).

7

Over a third of U.S. adults and seventeen percent of youth are obese

Obesity prevalence in the U.S. by age group (2009-2010)
Percent

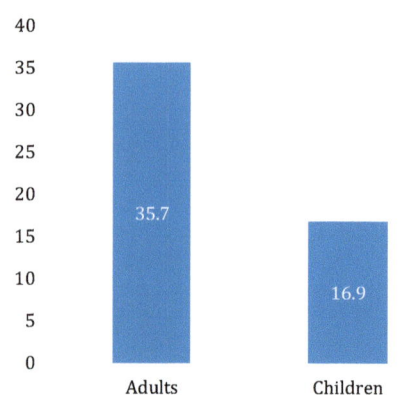

Obesity is defined as:
- Body Mass Index (BMI) of 30+ for adults (ages ≥ 20)
- BMI at or above the 95th percentile for age/ gender for children and adolescents (ages 2-19)

Source: Fryar et al. 2012. "Overweight and obesity statistics." http://win.niddk.nih.gov/publications/ PDFs/stat904z.pdf (accessed November 12, 2014).

8

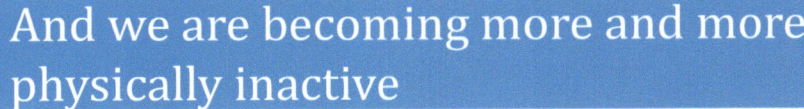

And we are becoming more and more physically inactive

Population reporting no leisure-time physical activity (1988-1994; 2009-2010)
Percent

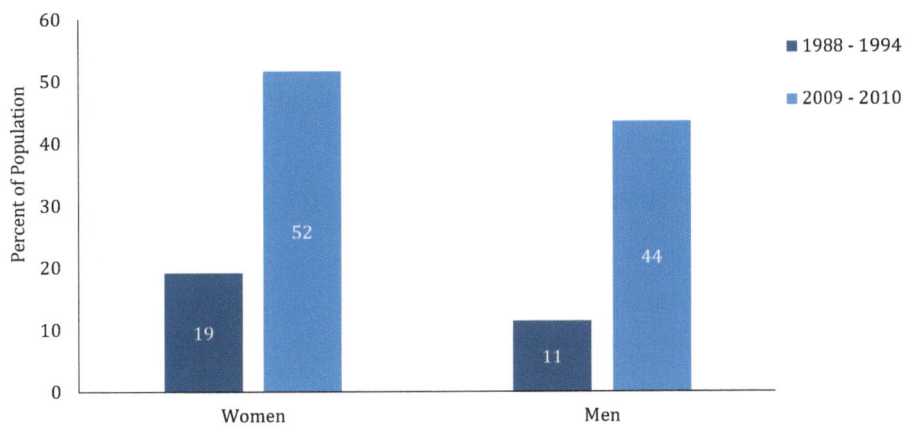

Source: Clark et al. 2013. "The healthiest regions in the United States." http://www.washingtonpost.com/wp-srv/special/health/us-life-expectancies/ (accessed August 14, 2014).

So how can we get the country back on track and begin to improve the health of the population?

Make the healthy choice, the default choice!

Implement comprehensive strategies to increase adherence to healthier behaviors through:

- **Environmental nudges** (e.g., create infrastructure conducive for walking and cycling; re-introduce physical education into schools)
- **Economic nudges** (e.g., change health benefit design; introduce "sin taxes")
- **Educational nudges** (e.g., leverage opinion leaders and/ or influential settings to promote health through education programs)

11

Moreover, start with nudges that promote physical activity (PA): PA "absolves other sins"

- **Environmental nudges**
  - Re-introduce exercise in schools (physical education classes, recess)
  - Create work environments that encourage people to walk 30 minutes per day
- **Economic nudges**
  - Vary health insurance premiums and/ or deductibles based on PA level, weight
  - Provide financial incentives for adhering to a PA regimen
- **Educational nudges**
  - Incorporate content around importance of PA into school curriculum
  - Leverage primary care office visits to educate patients on the importance of PA

12

Outline

1. Executive summary
2. The U.S. needs better health but healthcare delivery is not the answer
3. What has worked
4. Where to start

U.S. life expectancy lags behind the best of OECD nations

Japan (2013)	83.4 years
Spain (2013)	83.2 years
Switzerland (2013)	82.9 years
U.S. (2013)	78.8 years

- But life expectancy is a poor measure of the healthcare delivery system
- Life expectancy depends on many additional factors beyond healthcare delivery

Note: OECD= Organisation for Economic Co-operation and Development.
Source: OECD Health Statistics – Frequently Requested Data. July 2015. http://www.oecd.org/els/health-systems/oecd-health-statistics-2014-frequently-requested-data.htm (accessed July 14, 2015).

Sub-segments of U.S. population have the best life expectancy in the world...

Location	Life Expectancy (years)
Japan (2013)[1]	83.4
U.S. (2013)[1]	78.8
Los Angeles County Asian-Pacific Islander Americans (2006)[2]	84.8
Residents of Ross, California (2012)[3]	88.0

Source: 1. OECD Health Statistics – Frequently Requested Data. July 2015. http://www.oecd.org/els/health-systems/oecd-health-statistics-2014-frequently-requested-data.htm (accessed July 14, 2015); 2. Los Angeles County Department of Public Health. 2010. "Life Expectancy in Los Angeles County: How Long Do We Live and Why? A Cities and Communities Health Report." http://www.publichealth.lacounty.gov/epi/docs/Life%20Expectancy%20Final_web.pdf (accessed July 20, 2014); 3. Burd-Sharps, Sarah and Kristen Lewis. 2012. "A Portrait of Marin." *American Human Development Project of the Social Science Research Council.* http://www.measureofamerica.org/marin/ (accessed July 14, 2015).

While others are on par with developing nations, despite getting care in the same system

Location	Life Expectancy	
	Female (years)	Male (years)
Perry County, KY[1]	72.7	66.5
McDowell County, KY[1]	72.9	63.9
Algeria (2012)[2]	73.0	70.0

Source: 1. Clark et al. 2013. "The healthiest regions in the United States." *The Washington* Post. http://www.washingtonpost.com/wp-srv/special/health/us-life-expectancies/ (accessed July 30, 2014); 2. WHO. 2014. "Global Health Observatory Data Repository." http://apps.who.int /gho/data/view.main.60020?lang=en (accessed July 30, 2014).

Top 5 leading causes of death in the U.S. have a number of behavioral risk factors, e.g., tobacco use

Rank	Cause of Death (#)[1]	Risk Factors[2]
1	**Heart disease** (596,577)	*Tobacco use,* hypertension, high cholesterol, type 2 diabetes, *poor diet, overweight,* and *lack of physical activity.*
2	**Cancer** (576,691)	*Tobacco use, poor diet, lack of physical activity, overweight,* sun exposure, certain hormones, *alcohol,* some viruses and bacteria, ionizing radiation, and certain chemicals and other substances.
3	**Chronic lower respiratory diseases** (142,943)	*Tobacco smoke,* second-hand smoke exposure, other indoor air pollutants, outdoor air pollutants, allergens, and exposure to occupational agents.
4	**Stroke** (128,932)	Hypertension, high cholesterol, heart disease, diabetes, *overweight,* previous stroke, *tobacco use, alcohol use,* and *lack of physical activity.*
5	**Accidents** (126,438)	*Lack of seatbelt use, lack of motorcycle helmet use,* unsafe consumer products, *drug and alcohol use (including prescription drug misuse),* exposure to occupational hazards, and unsafe home and community environments.

Source: 1. Hoyert, Donna L and Jiaquan Xu. 2012. "Deaths: Preliminary data for 2011." *National Vital Statistics Report.* 61 (6): 1-52; 2. CDC. 2014. "Up to 40 percent of annual deaths from each of five leading US causes are preventable: Premature deaths from each cause due to modifiable risks." http://www.cdc.gov.ezproxy1.lib.asu.edu/media/releases/2014/p0501-preventable-deaths.html (accessed July 30, 2014).

Not surprisingly, more healthcare spending does not translate into increased longevity

Life expectancy at birth as a function of healthcare expenditures by country (2012 or nearest year)
Years

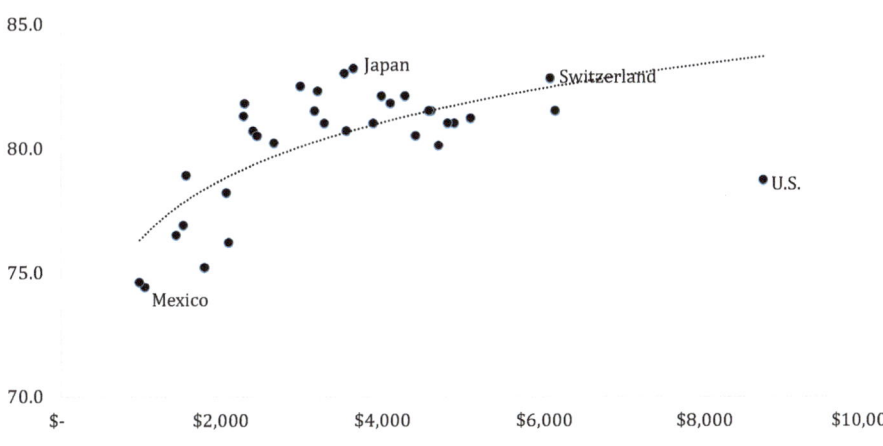

Source: OCED Health Statistics 2014 - Frequently Requested Data. 2014. http://www.oecd.org.ezproxy1.lib.asu.edu/els/health-systems/oecd-health-statistics-2014-frequently-requested-data.htm (accessed June 11, 2014).

Key behavioral culprits

- Tobacco use

- Obesity

- Physical inactivity

19

Tobacco use is still a major issue

- Smoking is the single most avoidable cause of disease, disability, and death in the United States
- Significant progress has been made in reducing the rate of smoking using environmental, economic, and educational approaches
- However, approximately one fifth of Americans still smoke

20

Smoking – "the persistent epidemic"

- Over the past 50 years (1964-2014) more than 20 million Americans died as a result of smoking, including
  - 2.5 million non-smokers
  - >100,000 babies
- Between 2010 and 2014, smoking was responsible for approximately
  - 90% of all lung cancer deaths
  - 61% of all pulmonary deaths
  - 32% of all coronary deaths

Source: U.S. Department of Health and Human Services. The Health Consequences of Smoking—50 Years of Progress. A Report of the Surgeon General. Atlanta, GA: U.S. Department of Health and Human Services, Centers for Disease Control and Prevention, National Center for Chronic Disease Prevention and Health Promotion, Office on Smoking and Health, 2014. Printed with corrections, January 2014. general-audience-presentation.ppt (accessed November 12, 2014).

Significant progress has been made, but >40 million Americans still smoke regularly

- The smoking rate has dropped by more than half over the past 50 years, from 43% in 1965 to a current rate of ~18%
- It is estimated that the reduction in smoking rates saved 8 million lives and added about 3 years to average life expectancy
- This progress has been attributed to a combination of approaches, including
  - Environmental, e.g., public space smoking bans
  - Economic, e.g., increasing the cost of cigarettes through taxation
  - Educational, e.g., public education media campaigns, package labeling

Source: U.S. Department of Health and Human Services. The Health Consequences of Smoking—50 Years of Progress. A Report of the Surgeon General. Atlanta, GA: U.S. Department of Health and Human Services, Centers for Disease Control and Prevention, National Center for Chronic Disease Prevention and Health Promotion, Office on Smoking and Health, 2014. Printed with corrections, January 2014. general-audience-presentation.ppt (accessed November 12, 2014).

Medical consequences of smoking are vast...

- Over the past 50 years cigarettes have become more deadly and more addictive
- Smoking causes disease in nearly every organ of the body, including
  - 13 different types of cancer
  - Chronic Obstructive Pulmonary Disease (COPD)
  - Cardiovascular disease
  - Blindness
- Moreover, secondhand smoke kills more than 41,000 nonsmokers every year, since it contains the same toxic ingredients inhaled by active smokers

Source: U.S. Department of Health and Human Services. The Health Consequences of Smoking—50 Years of Progress. A Report of the Surgeon General. Atlanta, GA: U.S. Department of Health and Human Services, Centers for Disease Control and Prevention, National Center for Chronic Disease Prevention and Health Promotion, Office on Smoking and Health, 2014. Printed with corrections, January 2014. general-audience-presentation.ppt (accessed November 12, 2014).

23

Further efforts to reduce smoking are warranted

- There is no safe level of secondhand smoke exposure, nor safe cigarettes
- Thus, additional efforts need to be directed at further reducing smoking prevalence in the population
- The good news is that we know what to do (e.g., smoke-free policies in public places), but a more concerted and comprehensive approach is warranted

Source: U.S. Department of Health and Human Services. The Health Consequences of Smoking—50 Years of Progress. A Report of the Surgeon General. Atlanta, GA: U.S. Department of Health and Human Services, Centers for Disease Control and Prevention, National Center for Chronic Disease Prevention and Health Promotion, Office on Smoking and Health, 2014. Printed with corrections, January 2014. general-audience-presentation.ppt (accessed November 12, 2014).

24

Key behavioral culprits

- Tobacco use

- Obesity

- Physical inactivity

25

Obesity rates have reached epidemic proportions

- The U.S. has one of the highest obesity rates in the world; obesity prevalence has been trending up for over 20 years
- Obesity is highly associated with the prevalence of one or more chronic diseases
- Children are an especially vulnerable population if overweight or obese early in life
- The health implications are projected to impact millions of Americans in the next two decades

Note: Obesity is defined as a body mass index (BMI) 30+

26

Whether self-reported or based on height and weight measures…

Obese population, self-reported (2013 or nearest year)
Percent total population

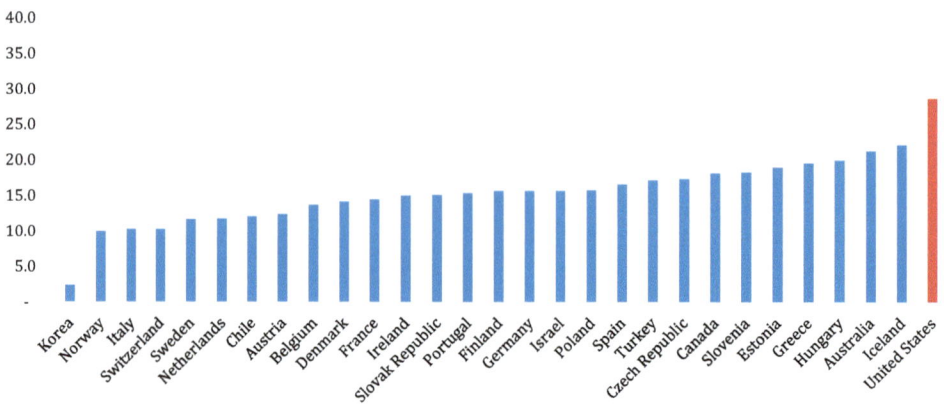

27

U.S. has one of the highest obesity rates among developed nations

Obese population, height and weight (2013 or nearest year)
Percent total population

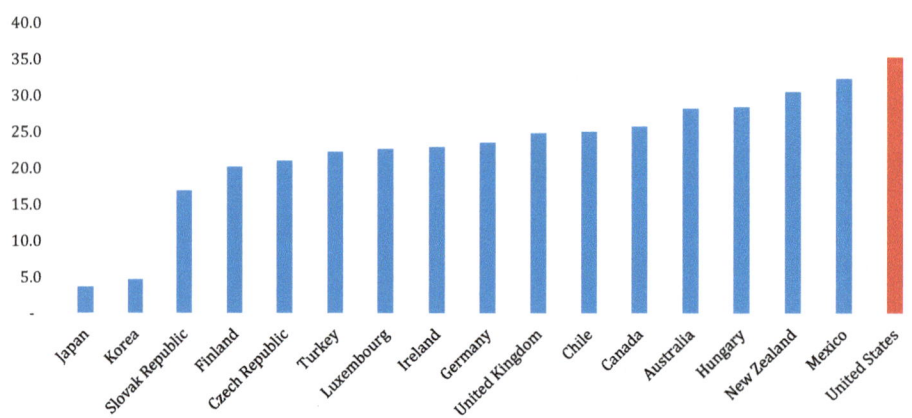

28

The prevalence of obesity in the U.S. has been on the rise over the past two decades

Percentage of U.S. adults who are obese (2011; BRFSS Methodology)

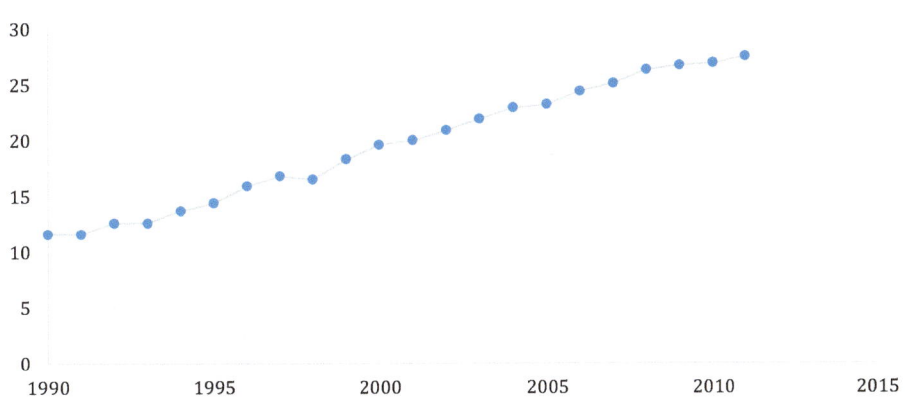

Note: BRFFS = Behavioral Risk Factor Surveillance System
Source: America's Health Rankings. Obesity: United states. 2014. http://www.americashealthrankings.org/ALL/Obesity (accessed November 11, 2014).

29

The medical consequences of obesity are vast

- Type 2 diabetes
- Heart disease
- High blood pressure
- Nonalcoholic fatty liver disease (excess fat and inflammation in the liver of people who drink little or no alcohol)
- Osteoarthritis (a health problem causing pain, swelling, and stiffness in one or more joints)
- Some types of cancer: breast, colon, endometrial (related to the uterine lining), and kidney
- Stroke

Source: Fryar et al. 2012. "Overweight and obesity statistics." In NIH Publications [database online]. Bethesda, MD. http://win.niddk.nih.gov/publications/PDFs/stat904z.pdf (accessed November 11, 2014).

30

Thus, projected trends are alarming

- "If states' obesity rates continue on their current trajectories, the number of new cases of type 2 diabetes, coronary heart disease and stroke, hypertension and arthritis could increase 10 times between 2010 and 2020 — and double again by 2030. Obesity could contribute to more than 6 million cases of type 2 diabetes, 5 million cases of coronary heart disease and stroke, and more than 400,000 cases of cancer in the next two decades."[1]

- In fact, Dr. Edward Gregg and his fellow researchers from the CDC have recently projected that 40% of Americans born between 2000–2011 will develop diabetes in their lifetime.[2]

Note: CDC= Centers for Disease Control and Prevention
Source: 1. Levi et al. 2013. "F as in fat: how obesity threatens America's future 2013." http://healthyamericans.org/assets/files/TFAH2013FasInFatReportFinal%209.9.pdf (accessed August 19, 2014).
2. Gregg et al. 2014. "Trends in lifetime risk and years of life lost due to diabetes in the USA, 1985-2011: a modelling study." *The Lancet Diabetes & Endocrinology*, early online publication. http://www.thelancet.com/journals/landia/article/PIIS2213-8587%2814%2970161-5/fulltext (accessed August 19, 2014).

Children are especially vulnerable; those overweight before the age of 5 are likely to be obese later in life

- 45% of children with obesity, between the ages of 5 and 14 years, were already overweight by the age of 5 years

- In comparison, only 13% of children who are normal weight in the eighth grade had been overweight in kindergarten

- Early onset overweight and obesity in children not only predisposes them to obesity later in life, it also predisposes them to risk factors for chronic diseases

Note: Overweight defined as a BMI at or above the 85th percentile and below the 95th percentile for children and teens of the same age and sex.
Source: Cunningham et al. 2014. "Incidence of childhood obesity in the United States." *New England Journal of Medicine*. 370 (5): 403-11.

Obese adolescents show higher prevalence of chronic disease risk factors than their normal weight peers

Prevalence of cardiovascular disease risk factors among U.S. adolescents (1999–2008, NHANES)
Percent

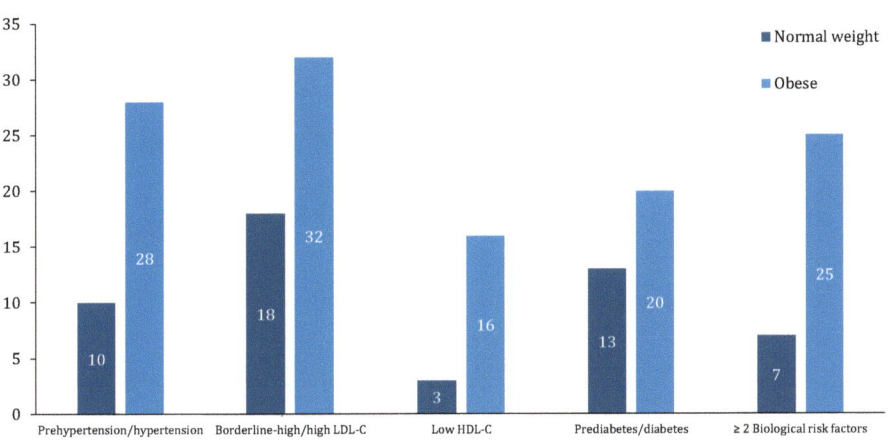

Note: NHANES = National Health and Nutrition Examination Survey
Source: May et al. 2012. "Prevalence of cardiovascular disease risk factors among US adolescents, 1999-2008." *Pediatrics*. 129 (6): 1035-41.

What is causing these trends?

A number of reports suggest that our overall calorie consumption has gone up, most likely as a result of:

- More calories being consumed outside the home[1]
- Growth in portion sizes[2]
- Increased consumption of sugar-sweetened beverages and highly processed sugars[3]

Source: 1. USDA. "Food-away-from-home." *United States Department of Agriculture: Economic Research Service.* http://www.ers.usda.gov/topics/food-choices-health/food-consumption-demand/food-away-from-home.aspx#.U3EqYS_Pp10 (accessed August 19, 2014); 2. Ghorayshi, A. 2012. "Too big to chug: How our sodas got so huge." http://www.motherjones.com/media/2012/06/supersize-biggest-sodas-mcdonalds-big-gulp-chart (accessed August 19, 2014); 3. Ervin, R Bethene and Cynthia L Ogden. 2013. "NCHS Data Brief: Consumption of Added Sugars Among U.S. Adults, 2005-2010." *Centers for Disease Control and Prevention.* http://www.cdc.gov/nchs/data/databriefs/db122.htm (accessed February 12, 2015).

In 2010, nearly half of personal food budgets were dedicated to meals and snacks prepared away from the home

Percent of personal food budget spent on meals and snacks prepared away from the home (1970-2010)

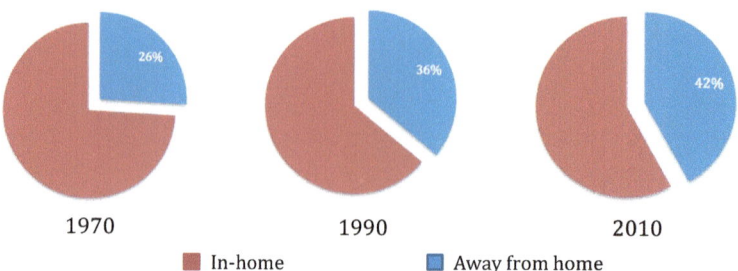

1970	1990	2010

■ In-home   ■ Away from home

"Frequently eating foods prepared away from home is associated with obesity, higher body fat and a higher BMI."

Source: USDA. "Food-away-from-home." *United States Department of Agriculture: Economic Research Service.* http://www.ers.usda.gov/topics/food-choices-health/food-consumption-demand/food-away-from-home.aspx#.U3EqYS_Pp10 (accessed August 19, 2014).

Moreover, the portion sizes have grown to astonishing amounts

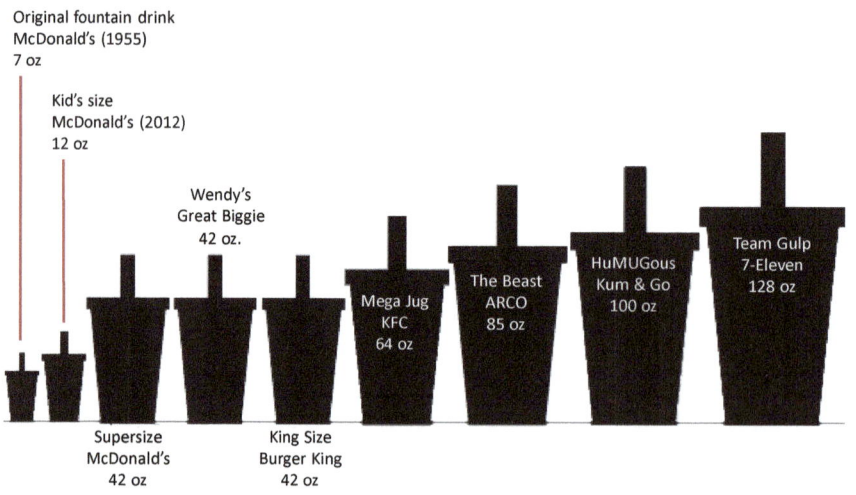

Original fountain drink
McDonald's (1955)
7 oz

Kid's size
McDonald's (2012)
12 oz

Wendy's
Great Biggie
42 oz.

Mega Jug
KFC
64 oz

The Beast
ARCO
85 oz

HuMUGous
Kum & Go
100 oz

Team Gulp
7-Eleven
128 oz

Supersize
McDonald's
42 oz

King Size
Burger King
42 oz

Source: Ghorayshi, A. 2012. "Too big to chug: How our sodas got so huge." http://www.motherjones.com/media/2012/06/supersize-biggest-sodas-mcdonalds-big-gulp-chart (accessed August 19, 2014); Photo credit: Soonerpa/flikr.

Some restaurants serve larger portions of the same product in the U.S. vs other countries

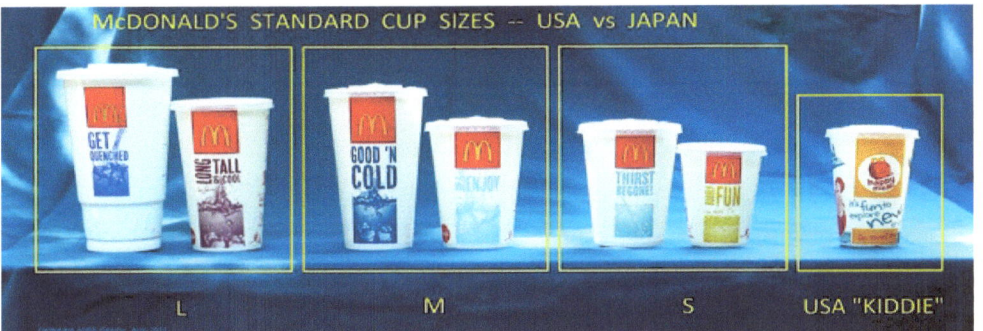

Source: Ghorayshi, A. 2012. "Too big to chug: How our sodas got so huge." http://www.motherjones.com/media/2012/06/supersize-biggest-sodas-mcdonalds-big-gulp-chart (accessed August 19, 2014);
Photo credit: Okinawa Soba/Flikr.

"Soft drinks…are the largest single source of calories in the American diet."[1]

Size	Source	Grams of Sugar[2]	Calories	Calories per oz
7 oz.	Original McDonald's ('55)	19.6	77	11
12 oz.	Kid's Size McDonald's ('12)	33.6	132	11
42 oz.	Supersize McDonald's	117.6	462	11
64 oz.	KFC	179.2	704	11
85 oz.	ARCO	238.0	935	11
100 oz.	Kum & Go	280.0	1100	11
128 oz.	7-Eleven Team Gulp	361.0	1408	11

Source: 1. Keystone Forum. 2006. *The keystone forum on away-from-home foods: Opportunities for preventing weight gain and obesity.* Washington, DC: The Keystone Center; 2. USDA. Basic report: 14400,
carbonated beverage, cola, contains caffeine, fast-food cola. 2014. http://ndb.nal.usda.gov/ndb/foods/show/4351?qlookup=14400&max= 25&man=&lfacet=&new=1 (accessed December 19, 2014) .

The U.S. comes in second only to Argentina in global soda consumption

Top 10 soda drinking countries in the world, 2014
Soft drink purchases per capita, in liters

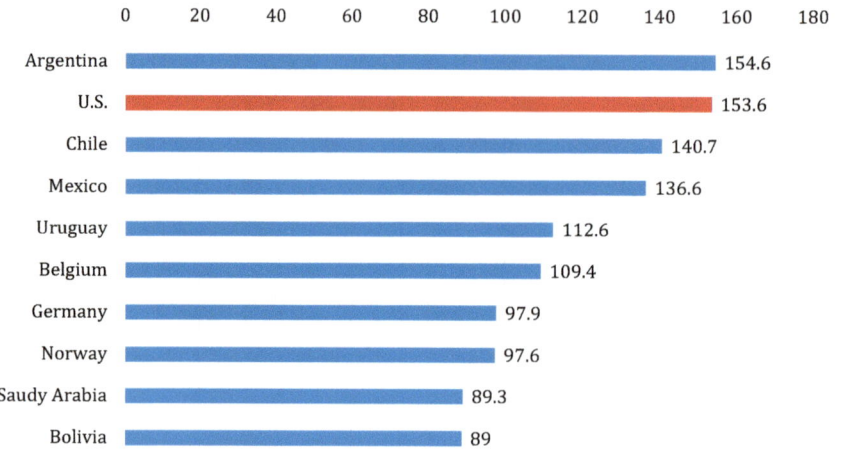

Source: Silver, M. 2015. "I'd like to buy the emerging world a Coke". http://www.npr.org/sections/goatsandsoda/2015/05/20/408027045/id-like-to-buy-the-emerging-world-a-coke (accessed on July 18, 2015).

In fact, average daily consumption of added sugars far exceeds the recommended daily allowance set by the WHO and the American Heart Association

Recommended daily allowance vs. average daily kilocalories consumed from added sugars among U.S. adults, aged 20+ (2005-2010)

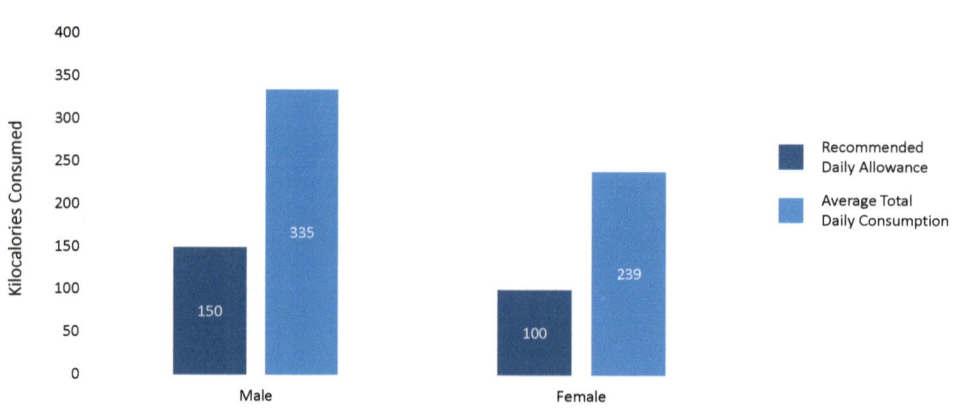

Source: 1. Guideline: Sugars intake for adults and children. Geneva: World Health Organization; 2015; 2. AHA. 2014. "Added Sugars." *American Health Association.* http://www.heart.org/HEARTORG/GettingHealthy/NutritionCenter/HealthyEating/Added-Sugars_UCM_305858_Article.jsp (accessed February 12, 2015); 3. Ervin, R Bethene and Cynthia L Ogden. "NCHS Data Brief: Consumption of Added Sugars Among U.S. Adults, 2005-2010." *Centers for Disease Control and Prevention.* 2013. http://www.cdc.gov/nchs/data/databriefs/db122.htm (accessed February 12, 2015).

Key behavioral culprits

- Tobacco use

- Obesity

- Physical inactivity

41

Physical inactivity

- Less than half of Americans meet the recommended physical activity guidelines
- Both leisure and occupational activities have been decreasing steadily
- The majority of schools fail to provide daily physical education to students
- Physical inactivity increases risk of preventable chronic diseases and mortality

42

Physical activity guidelines for adults (ages 18-64)

- Moderate-intensity aerobic activity (e.g., brisk walking)
  - 150 minutes per week or
  - 30 minutes per day, 5 days per week
- Muscle strengthening activities that work all major muscle groups, i.e., legs, hips, back, abdomen, chest, shoulders, and arms
  - 2 times per week

Source: CDC. 2014. "Facts about physical activity." http://www.cdc.gov.ezproxy1.lib.asu.edu/physicalactivity/data/facts.html (accessed August 11, 2014).

So how do we measure up?

- Only 48% of U.S. adults meet the guidelines for aerobic activity,[1] and
- Only 20% meet the guidelines for both aerobic and muscle-strengthening activities[2]

Source: 1. CDC. 2014. "Facts about physical activity." http://www.cdc.gov.ezproxy1.lib.asu.edu/physicalactivity/data/facts.html (accessed August 11, 2014); 2. CDC. 2014."Health, United States, 2013: With special feature on prescription drugs." *U.S. Department of Health and Human Services.*

And we are becoming more and more physically inactive

Population reporting no leisure-time physical activity (1988-1994; 2009-2010)
Percent

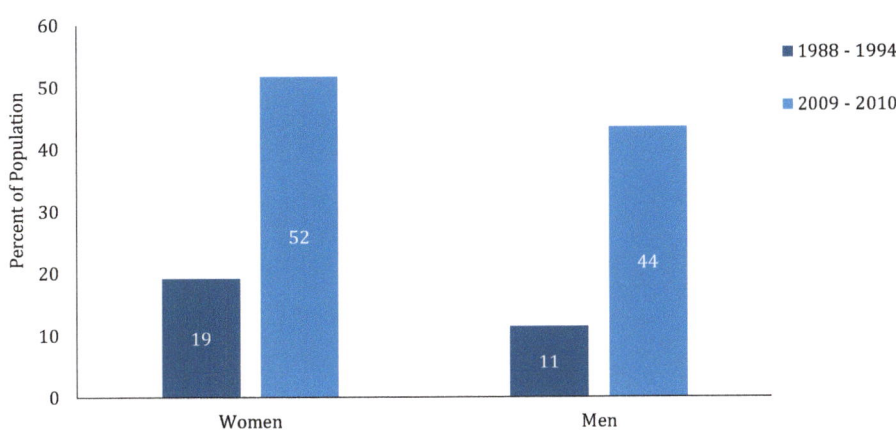

Source: Clark et al. 2013. "The healthiest regions in the United States." Available from http://www.washingtonpost.com/wp-srv/special/health/us-life-expectancies/ (accessed August 14, 2014).

Occupational activity is also declining

Traditional Amish farmers average[1]:

- 16,311 steps/day
- 41 hours/week of physical activity
- 4.5% obesity rate

Modern American workers average[2]:

- 5,117 steps/day
- 2 hours/week of physical activity[3]
- 34% obesity rate

We have also cut back on physical activity required to get to and from work, "Today, a mere 2 percent of us walk to work...ten times less than fifty years ago."[4]

Source: 1. Bassett et al. 2004. "Physical activity in an old order Amish community." *Journal of the American College of Sports Medicine.* 36(1): 79-85; 2. Basset et al. 2010. "Pedometer-measured physical activity and health behaviors in U.S. adults." *Journal of the American College of Sports Medicine.* 2010. 42(10): 1819-25; 3. Messer, A. 2012. "Americans fall short of federal exercise recommendations." http://news.psu.edu/story/149052/2012/05/08/americans-fall-short-federal-exercise-recommendations (accessed November 11, 2014); 4. Levine, James and Selene Yeager. 2009. "Move a little, lose a lot: new N.E.A.T. science reveals how to be thinner, happier and smarter." p.15. New York, NY: Crown Publishers.

Physical activity guidelines for children (<18 years of age)

- Moderate intensity physical activity (e.g., brisk walking)
  - 420 minutes per week or
  - 60 minutes per day, every day
- Included in this should be body-weight muscle strengthening activities and bone strengthening activities (e.g., push-ups, jumping, running)

Source: CDC. 2011. "How much physical activity do children need?" http://www.cdc.gov.ezproxy1.lib.asu.edu/physicalactivity/everyone/guidelines/children.html (accessed November 11, 2014).

Less than a third of students in grades 9-12 meet physical activity guidelines

Adolescents who were **not** physically active at least 60 min per day on all 7 days, by grade (2013)
Percent

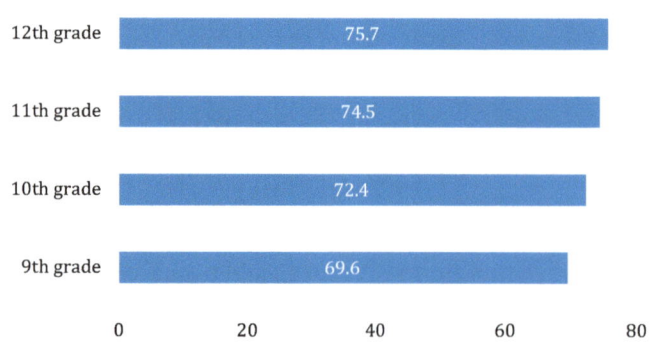

Source: Healthy People 2020. 2014. "Meeting guidelines for aerobic physical activity, adolescents, 2011." http://www.healthypeople.gov/2020/topics-objectives/topic/physical-activity/national-snapshot?topicId=33 (accessed December 19, 2014).

The majority of schools in the U.S. fail to provide daily physical education for students

Percentage of U.S. schools providing daily physical education (2006)

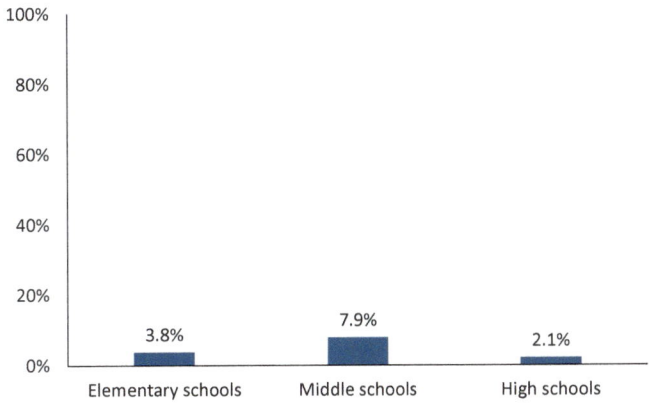

This is predominantly based upon the argument that physical education takes away from time and resources that should be allocated to math, reading, and sciences.

Source: Trost, S. 2007. "Active education: physical education, physical activity, and academic performance." *Active Living Research*, 1-5.

Where has all the play gone in schools?

- In 2001, the No Child Left Behind act required schools to meet strict reading, mathematics, and science performance scores in order to receive funding
- Elementary schools responded by:

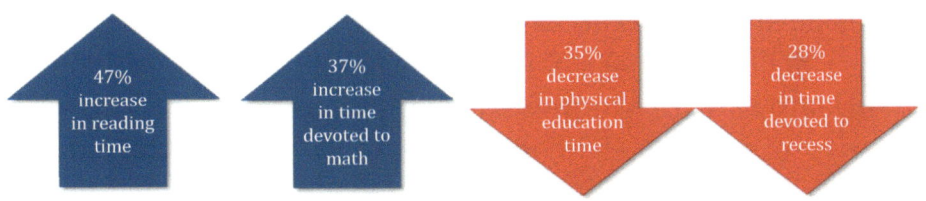

Source: Franklin, S. 2011. "Facts: Physical activity promotion in education." *National Coalition for Promoting Physical Activity*. ttp://ncppa.org/static/assets/NPAP_Fact_Sheet-Education.pdf (accessed August 19, 2014).

This is very unfortunate given the many benefits associated with physical activity in children

- "...adding time to 'academic' or 'curricular' subjects by taking time from physical education programmes does not enhance grades in these subjects and may be detrimental to health."[1]

- In fact, extracurricular activities, like sports or curricular physical education, "are likely to increase attachment to school and self-esteem which are indirect but important factors in academic achievement."[1]

- "Adolescents who reported either participating in school activities, such as physical education and team sports, or playing sports with their parents, were 20 percent more likely than their sedentary peers to earn an "A" in math or English."[2]

Source: 1. Trudeau, Francois and Roy Shephard. 2009. "Physical education, school physical activity, school sports and academic performance." *International Journal of Behavioral Nutrition and Physical Activity.* 5 (10); 2. Trost, S. 2007. "Active education: Physical education, physical activity, and academic performance." *Active Living Research*, 1-5.

Lack of physical activity has significant morbidity and mortality implications

- Prolonged sitting has been shown to double the risk of metabolic syndrome – a precursor to heart disease and diabetes[1]

- A study tracking the health of 123,000 Americans between 1992 and 2006 showed that[2]
  - Men who spent 6 hours or more per day of their leisure time sitting had an overall death rate that was about 20% higher than the men who sat for 3 hours or less
  - Death rate for women who sat for more than 6 hours a day was about 40% higher than the women who sat for 3 hours of less

Source: 1. Levine, James and Selene Yeager. 2009. "Move a little, lose a lot: new N.E.A.T. science reveals how to be thinner, happier and smarter." p.27. New York, NY: Crown Publishers; 2. Vlahos, J. 2011. "Is sitting a lethal activity?" *The New York Times.* http://www.nytimes.com/2011/04/17/magazine/mag-17sitting-t.html?_r=0. (accessed November 12, 2014).

Outline

1. Executive summary
2. The U.S. needs better health but healthcare delivery is not the answer
3. **What has worked**
4. Where to start

- Studies suggest that
  - Sticking with a healthier plan of action is more important than the details of that plan
  - Nudging, i.e., interventions that rely less on conscious choice by individuals and more on surrounding environment/societal norms are more likely to succeed
- Thus, we need to find ways to make the healthy choice, the default choice

Long-term adherence to a diet is far more important than the type of diet

- The variance in weight-loss and reduced risk of diseases between various diets including low-carbohydrate, low-fat, and Mediterranean diets has proven to be small and inconsistent[1,2]

- However, regardless of which diet is followed, clinically significant weight-loss is seen among those who adhere to their diet of choice[1,2]

Source: 1. Johnston et al. 2014. "Comparison of Weight Loss Among Named Diet Programs in Overweight and Obese Adults." *JAMA*, 312(9):923-933; 2. Pagoto, Sherry L and Bradley M Appelhans. 2013. "A Call for an End to the Diet Debates." *JAMA*, 310(7):687-688.

The same conclusions seem to apply to physical activity

- Those who are of normal weight, or have successfully battled obesity, adhere to a more physically active lifestyle [1,2]

- 94% of those who successfully lose weight increase their overall physical activity levels[2]

Source: 1. Johnston et al. 2014. "Comparison of Weight Loss Among Named Diet Programs in Overweight and Obese Adults." *JAMA*, 312(9):923-933; 2. Pagoto, Sherry L and Bradley M Appelhans. 2013. "A Call for an End to the Diet Debates." *JAMA*, 310(7):687-688.

Nudging example: Opt-out program for organ donation vastly increases donation rates

- Organ donation opt-in
  - Donors must declare that they do indeed want to be an organ donor
  - Germany uses this approach where about 12% of the population are currently consenting organ donors
- Organ donation opt-out
  - Based on the notion of presumed consent, all citizens are considered consenting donors unless they declare otherwise
  - Austria uses this approach where about 99% of the population are currently consenting organ donors
- Similar strategies can be utilized to modulate health behaviors

Source: Thaler, R. 2009. "Opting in vs. Opting out." *The New York Times*. http://www.nytimes.com/2009/09/27/business/economy /27view.html (accessed September 3, 2014).

Make the healthy choice, the default choice by employing "nudging" techniques

Implement comprehensive strategies to increase adherence to healthier behaviors through

- Environmental nudges
- Economic nudges
- Educational nudges

The built environment matters...

- "Transportation infrastructure—public transit, greenways and trails, sidewalks and safe street crossings near schools, bicycle paths, traffic–calming devices, and sidewalks that connect schools and homes to destinations—are associated with more walking and bicycling, greater physical activity and lower obesity rates."[1]
- "Participants with poor access to recreational facilities [have] a 68% greater chance of being obese."[2]

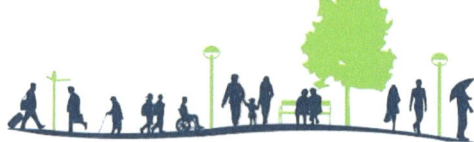

Source: 1. Rodriguez, D. 2009. "Active transportation: making the link from transportation to physical activity and obesity." *Active Living Research Report Brief*; 2. Booth et al. 2005. "Obesity and the built environment." *Journal of the American Dietetic Association*, 105(5S), 110-117. http://files.kff.org/attachment/2014-employer-health-benefits-survey-full-report (accessed December 3, 2014).

Evidence suggests that walking and biking to and from work is correlated with lower obesity rates

Adults self-reporting as obese by state (2007)
Percent

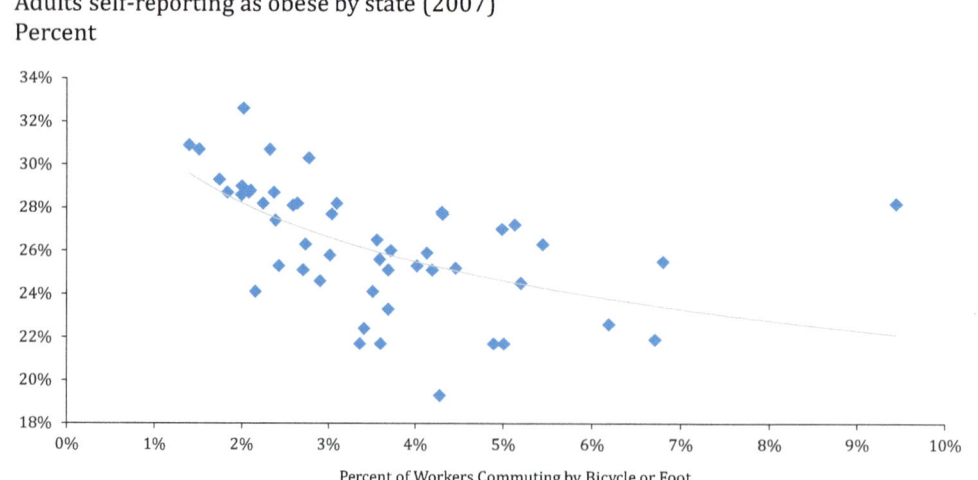

Percent of Workers Commuting by Bicycle or Foot

Source: Pucher et al. 2010. "Walking and cycling to health: a comparative analysis of city, state, and international data." *American Journal of Public Health*, 100(10):1986-1992.

Where you spend most of your day matters...

- The majority of U.S. adults spend a significant and increasing portion of their day at work; thus worksites provide opportunities for health interventions[1,2]

- A similar statement maybe made about the student population; thus school environments provide ideal settings for health interventions[2,3]

Source: 1. Milani, Richard V and Carl J Lavie. 2009. "Impact of worksite wellness intervention on cardiac risk factors and one-year health care costs." *American Journal of Cardiology*, 104:1389-1392; 2. Bureau of Labor Statistics. 2014. "American time U.S. survey." http://www.bls.gov/tus/charts/ (accessed December 3, 2014); 3. Swanbrow, D. 2004. "U.S. children and teens spend more time on academics." http://www.ur.umich.edu/0405/Dec06_04/20.shtml (accessed December 3, 2014).

Smoke-free policies in the workplace have been shown to reduce tobacco use

- A 100% smoke-free worksite leads to a 23% reduction in smoking prevalence and 14% lower average daily cigarette consumption among smokers; partial bans diminish both types of impact

- Greatest impact was observed in groups/ industries with the highest smoking prevalence and daily cigarette consumption

Sources: Farrelly et al. 1999. "The impact of workplace smoking bans: results from a national survey." *Tobacco Control*, 8:272-277.

Smoke-free policies in the workplace have been shown to reduce tobacco use cont'd

- A systematic review of 26 studies on smoke-free workplaces across 4 countries showed that in 100% smoke-free environments, the combined effect of lower prevalence and lower consumption resulted in a 29% reduction in tobacco use

- "To obtain the 29% drop in employee consumption resulting from smoke-free workplaces would require an increase in the price of cigarettes of 73%."

Sources: Fichtenberg, Caroline M and Stanton A Glantz. 2002. "Effect of smoke-free workplaces on smoking behavior: systematic review." *BMJ*, 325:1-7.

Most employers also offer at least one worksite wellness program...

Firms offering a particular wellness program to their employees, by firm size (2014)
Percentage

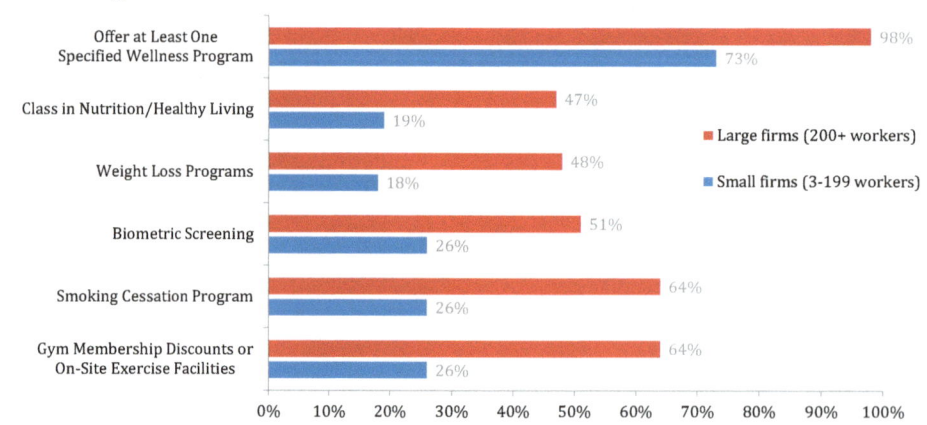

Note: Data reflective only of firms offering health benefits. Biometric screening is a health examination that measures an employee's risk factors such as cholesterol, blood pressure, stress, and nutrition.

Source: Claxton et al. 2014. "Employer Health Benefits: 2014 Annual Survey." *The Kaiser Family Foundation and Health Research and Educational Trust.*

Worksite wellness programs show positive impacts on employee health...

Although, the designs and evaluation of the various worksite wellness programs are highly variable, the results show generally positive trends, e.g.,

- A 6-months comprehensive worksite wellness program focused on cardiac risk factors showed significant improvements in employee health risk status, with 57% of high-risk employees converting to low-risk status[1]

- A worksite program that encouraged employees to achieve 10,000 daily steps has resulted in improved blood pressure control and weight loss[2]

Source: 1. Milani, Richard V and Carl J Lavie. 2009. "Impact of worksite wellness intervention on cardiac risk factors and one-year health care costs." *American Journal of Cardiology*, 104:1389-1392; 2. Carnethon et al. 2009. "Worksite wellness programs for cardiovascular disease prevention: a policy statement from the American Heart Association. *Circulation*, 120:1725-1741.

...and employer bottom line

- Analysis of wellness programs provided by large employers showed that average employer medical costs fell $3.27 for every dollar spent on wellness programs

- Across employers of all sizes, worksite health promotion programs have been shown to result in ~ 25% reduction in sick leave, health insurance costs, as well as workers compensation and disability costs

Source: James, J. 2013. "Health policy brief: workplace wellness programs." *Health Affairs*. http://healthaffairs.org/healthpolicybriefs/brief_pdfs/healthpolicybrief_93.pdf (accessed December 4, 2014).

The school environment offers a number of nudging levers to impact the health of our youth

- Re-instate physical education
  - 60 minutes/day of exercise time in schools results in a 14% reduced risk of becoming obese among school-aged kids

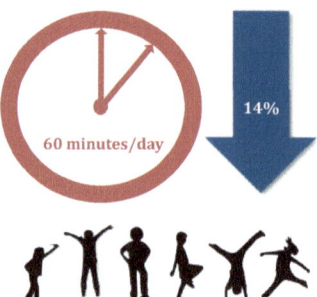

Source: 1. Cawley et al. 2013. "The impact of physical education on obesity among elementary school children." *Journal of Health Economics*, 32:743-755; 2. Seo and Lee. 2012. "Association of school nutrition policy and parental control with childhood overweight." *Journal of School Health*, 82(6): 285-293; 3. Whitmore-Schanzenbach, D. 2009. "Do School Lunches Contribute to Childhood Obesity." *Journal of Human Resources*, 44(3):684-709.

The school environment offers a number of nudging levers to impact the health of our youth

- Limit access to unhealthy snacks
  - "Children who attend schools where soda pop and non-low fat salty snacks could be purchased were more likely to be obese than those at school where such items were not sold."

Source: Whitmore-Schanzenbach, D. 2009. "Do School Lunches Contribute to Childhood Obesity." *Journal of Human Resources*, 44(3):684-709.

The school environment offers a number of nudging levers to impact the health of our youth

- Implement higher nutritional standards in school lunch programs
  - Students who regularly eat school lunches are 29% more likely to be obese than those who eat a lunch made at home[1]
  - In fact, "as few as 40 additional calories per day could lead to a two percentage point difference in obesity rates among children." [2]

Source: 1. Eagle et al. 2010. "Health Status and behavior among middle-school children in a mid-west community: what are the underpinnings of childhood obesity?" *American Heart Journal*, 160(6):1185-1189; 2. Whitmore-Schanzenbach, D. 2009. "Do School Lunches Contribute to Childhood Obesity." *Journal of Human Resources*, 44(3): 684-709.

The social environment matters...

- You are at an increased risk of smoking, obesity, and alcohol consumption when your closest peers smoke, are obese, or consume alcohol

- However, healthy choices can also be extremely contagious: If that same peer quits smoking, we are 36% more likely to quit smoking ourselves

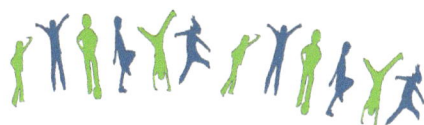

Source: Christakis, Nicholas A and James H Fowler. 2013. "Social contagion theory: examining dynamic social networks and human behavior." *Statistics in Medicine*, 32:556-577.

Research shows that social ties are highly predictive of our health behaviors

Increased likelihood of smoking, obesity, and alcohol consumption when closest peers smoke, are obese, or consume alcohol

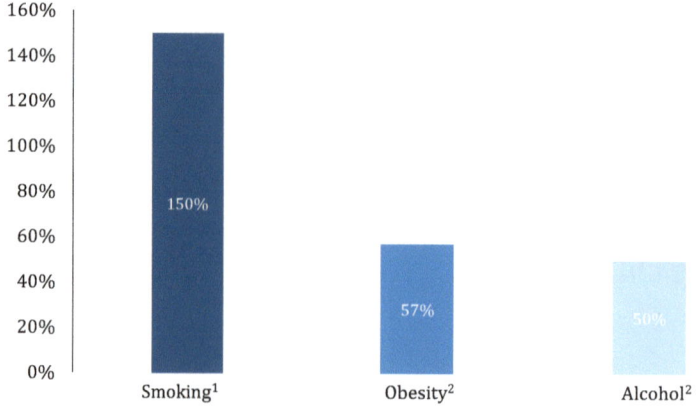

Source: Ball et al. 2010. "Is healthy behavior contagious: associations of social norms with physical activity and healthy eating." *International Journal of Behavioral Nutrition and Physical Activity*, 7:86; 2. Rofling, K. 2011. "Good health is contagious: power of social media spreads healthy lifestyle." *CDCH Solutions*. January/February: 35-37.

Which yields tremendous opportunity to spread healthier behavior choices among peer groups

- The Alliance for a Healthier Minnesota in collaboration with RedBrick Health demonstrated the power of utilizing social networks to promote physical activity
- Employees were invited "to participate in team-based weight loss, physical activity and nutrition challenges over three months."
- 10,000 employees from Blue Cross and Blue Shield of Minnesota, Cargill, General Mills, HealthPartners, Medtronic, Target and UnitedHealth Group partook in the Challenge—competing with teams within their office, while concurrently competing against the other companies
- The results?
  - 37,000 lbs. lost and 16.5 million minutes of activity logged

Source: Rofling, K. 2011. "Good health is contagious: power of social media spreads healthy lifestyle." *CDCH Solutions*. January/February: 35-37.

Make the healthy choice, the default choice by employing "nudging" techniques

Implement comprehensive strategies to increase adherence to healthier behaviors through

- Environmental nudges
- Economic nudges
- Educational nudges

Economic incentives provide another great nudging lever

- **"Sin taxes"** serve as a behavioral "user fee" that attempts to recover the costs of some of the externalities associated with unhealthy behaviors[1-3]

- **Employee health benefit plans** that incorporate economic incentives to influence behavior choices have shown positive results[4]

- **Social benefit plans** may offer an additional point of influence

Source: 1. CDC. 2010. "State cigarette excise taxes: United States 2009." *Morbidity and Mortality Weekly Report*, 59(13):385-388; 2. Marr, Chuck and Chye-Ching Huang. 2014. "Higher tobacco taxes can improve health and raise revenue." *Center on Budget and Policy Priorities.* http://www.cbpp.org/cms/index.cfm?fa=view&id=3978 (accessed on November 12, 2014); 3. Wagenaar et al. 2010. "Effects of alcohol tax and price policies on morbidity and mortality: a systematic review." *American Journal of Public Health*, 100(11):2270-2278; 4. Kelleher, D. "Live life, live long, live well: an evolving health and wellness strategy." Presented at Consumer-Centric Health Models for Change 2011 Conference, Seattle, October 13, 2011.

Sin taxes can address major drivers of poor health: Smoking

- A 10% increase in cigarette prices translates to a 4% reduction in consumption[1]
- This impact is even greater among groups that are typically more difficult to reach through public health programs – especially the young and the poor as they "are particularly sensitive to price increases."[2]

Source: 1. CDC. 2010. "State cigarette excise taxes: United States 2009." *Morbidity and Mortality Weekly Report*, 59(13):385-388; 2. Marr, Chuck and Chye-Ching Huang. 2014. "Higher tobacco taxes can improve health and raise revenue." *Center on Budget and Policy Priorities.* http://www.cbpp.org/cms/index.cfm?fa=view&id=3978 (accessed on November 12, 2014).

The price of cigarettes directly impacts cigarette sales

Cigarette sales and average price per pack in the U.S. (1970–2012)*

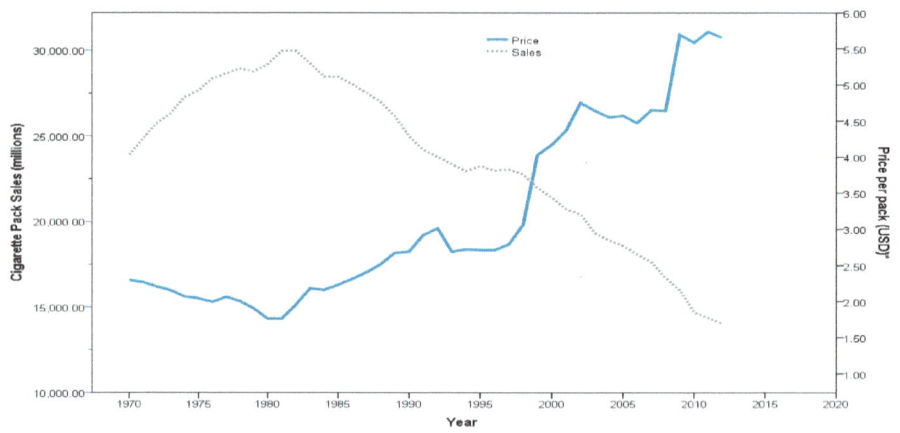

*Adjusted to 2012 dollars.

Source: The Tax Burden On Tobacco: Historical Compilation, 2012. Volume 47.

Price increases are approximately 2X as effective at reducing smoking among youth and greatly impact health among the poor

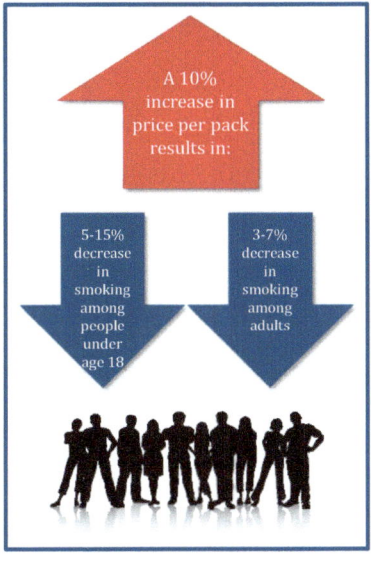

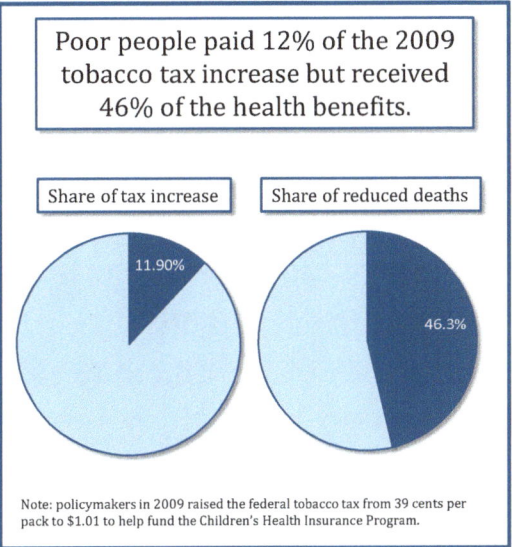

Poor people paid 12% of the 2009 tobacco tax increase but received 46% of the health benefits.

Share of tax increase — 11.90%

Share of reduced deaths — 46.3%

Note: policymakers in 2009 raised the federal tobacco tax from 39 cents per pack to $1.01 to help fund the Children's Health Insurance Program.

Source: Marr, Chuck and Chye-Ching Huang. 2014. "Higher tobacco taxes can improve health and raise revenue." *Center on Budget and Policy Priorities.* http://www.cbpp.org/cms/index.cfm?fa=view&id=3978 (accessed on November 12, 2014).

Sin taxes can address major drivers of poor health: Unhealthy nutrition habits

- Sugar Sweetened Beverages are responsible for significant morbidity and mortality in many countries[1]
- The U.S. comes in second worldwide in soda consumption[2]
- Modeling suggests a 1 cent per ounce tax on sugar sweetened beverages in the US could reduce consumption by ~20%[3]
- Preliminary results from Mexico show reductions in soda purchases of 6-12% within a year of implementing a 10% "soda tax"[4]

Source: 1. Singh et al. 2015. "Estimated global, regional, and national disease burdens related to sugar-sweetened beverage consumption in 2010." *Circulation*, doi: 10.1161/CIRCULATIONAHA.114.010636; 2. Silver, M. 2015. "I'd like to buy the emerging world a Coke". http://www.npr.org/sections/goatsandsoda/2015/05/20/408027045/id-like-to-buy-the-emerging-world-a-coke (accessed on July 18, 2015); 3. Andreyeva et al. 2011. "Estimating the potential of taxes on sugar-sweetened beverages to reduce consumption and generate revenue." *Preventive Medicine*, 52 (2011) 413–416; 4. Barclay, E. 2015. "Mexico's sugary drink tax makes a dent in consumption, study claims". http://www.npr.org/sections/thesalt/2015/06/19/415741354/mexicos-sugary-drink-tax-makes-a-dent-in-consumption-study-claims (accessed on July 18, 2015).

Economic incentives provide another great nudging lever

- **"Sin taxes"** serve as a behavioral "user fee" that attempts to recover the costs of some of the externalities associated with unhealthy behaviors[1-3]

- **Employee health benefit plans** that incorporate economic incentives to influence behavior choices have shown positive results[4]

- **Social benefit plans** may offer an additional point of influence

Source: 1. CDC. 2010. "State cigarette excise taxes: United States 2009." *Morbidity and Mortality Weekly Report*, 59(13):385-388; 2. Marr, Chuck and Chye-Ching Huang. 2014. "Higher tobacco taxes can improve health and raise revenue." *Center on Budget and Policy Priorities*. http://www.cbpp.org/cms/index.cfm?fa=view&id=3978 (accessed on November 12, 2014); 3. Wagenaar et al. 2010. "Effects of alcohol tax and price policies on morbidity and mortality: a systematic review." *American Journal of Public Health*, 100(11):2270-2278; 4. Kelleher, D. "Live life, live long, live well: an evolving health and wellness strategy." Presented at Consumer-Centric Health Models for Change 2011 Conference, Seattle, October 13, 2011.

Incentives embedded into employer health benefit plans provide another lever to impact behavior

- In 2005, 74% of the total health care costs for Safeway could be attributed to the prevalence of cardiovascular disease, cancer, diabetes, and obesity among employees
- To address these issues, Safeway developed a rebate and incentive plan to control risk factors for these conditions, specifically
    - Employees received reductions to medical benefit premiums if they were able to:
        - ✓ Refrain from smoking
        - ✓ Maintain a BMI below 30
        - ✓ Show no signs of hypertension
        - ✓ Sustain healthy ranges of cholesterol and blood glucose levels
    - Those who missed one or more of the goals had the opportunity to earn retroactive rebates if they improved sufficiently by year end

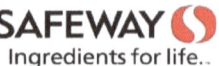

SAFEWAY
Ingredients for life..

Source: Kelleher, D. "Live life, live long, live well: an evolving health and wellness strategy." Presented at Consumer-Centric Health Models for Change 2011 Conference, Seattle, October 13, 2011.

Five years after implementation of the rebate and incentive plan, positive improvements were seen across all health metrics

Percentage of Safeway employees that moved from unhealthy to healthy status, by health indicator (2005-2010)

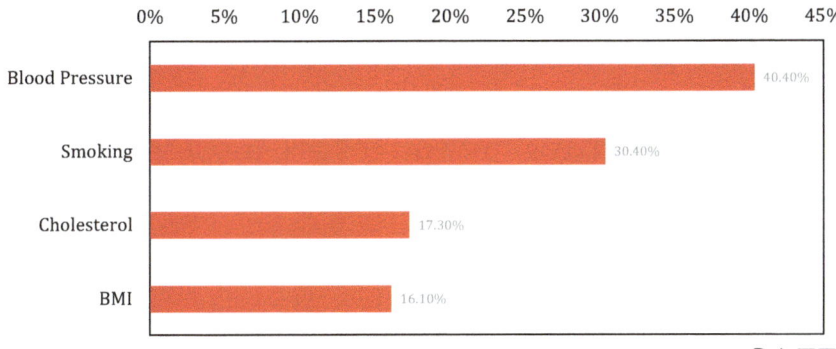

Source: Kelleher, D. "Live life, live long, live well: an evolving health and wellness strategy." Presented at Consumer-Centric Health Models for Change 2011 Conference, Seattle, October 13, 2011.

In fact, many other companies now include incentives in their health benefits offerings

- A 2011 survey of large employers found that ~50% already employ or plan to implement financial penalties (primarily through higher insurance premiums) for employees who do not participate in wellness programs[1]
- A 2013 RAND Employer Survey showed 31% of employers administer financial incentives through their group health plans[2]
  - These incentives were tied to participation in wellness programs and/ or achievement of health-related standards
  - Tobacco use was the primary behavior targeted with financial incentives tied to a health standard
  - In this employer sample, incentives were typically administered as rewards, with 84% of employers reporting the use of rewards, rather than penalties

Source: 1. James, J. 2013. "Health policy brief: workplace wellness programs." *Health Affairs,* http://healthaffairs.org/healthpolicybriefs/brief_pdfs/ healthpolicybrief_93.pdf (accessed December 4, 2014); 2. Mattke et al. 2013. "Workplace wellness programs study: final report." *RAND Health.* http://www.rand.org/content/dam/rand/pubs/research_reports/RR200/RR254/RAND_RR254.pdf (accessed November 4, 2014).

"To inform both the financial and policy questions... researchers, along with other behavioral and health sciences experts across the country, continue to focus on what size and what form of incentives are most likely to evoke and sustain health actions and behavior change."

Source: Terry, Paul and David R Anderson. 2012. "The role of incentives in improving engagement and outcomes in population health management: an evidenced-based perspective." *StayWell Health Management*. http://staywell.com/wp-content/uploads/2012/11/StayWell-Health-Management-incentives-white-paper.pdf (accessed January 26, 2015).

Economic incentives provide another great nudging lever

- **"Sin taxes"** serve as a behavioral "user fee" that attempts to recover the costs of some of the externalities associated with unhealthy behaviors[1-3]

- **Employee health benefit plans** that incorporate economic incentives to influence behavior choices have shown positive results[4]

- **Social benefit plans** may offer an additional point of influence

Source: 1. CDC. 2010. "State cigarette excise taxes: United States 2009." *Morbidity and Mortality Weekly Report*, 59(13):385-388; 2. Marr , Chuck and Chye-Ching Huang. 2014. "Higher tobacco taxes can improve health and raise revenue." *Center on Budget and Policy Priorities*. http://www.cbpp.org/cms/index.cfm?fa=view&id=3978 (accessed on November 12, 2014); 3. Wagenaar et al. 2010. "Effects of alcohol tax and price policies on morbidity and mortality: a systematic review." *American Journal of Public Health*, 100(11):2270-2278; 4. Kelleher, D. "Live life, live long, live well: an evolving health and wellness strategy." Presented at Consumer-Centric Health Models for Change 2011 Conference, Seattle, October 13, 2011.

The SNAP program provides a potential point intervention

- Studies have found that "SNAP participants' consumption was significantly sensitive to SNAP benefit changes and food price variations."

- Moreover, a recent study by Basu et al. suggests that placing a ban on using SNAP dollars to buy sugar sweetened beverages (SSB's) would not only lead to reduced consumption, but would also be expected to significantly reduce obesity prevalence and type-II diabetes among SNAP participants

Note: SNAP = Supplemental Nutrition Assistance Program
Source: Basu et al. 2014. "Ending SNAP subsidies for sugar sweetened beverages could reduce obesity and type 2 diabetes. *Health Affairs*, (6):1032-1039.

The WIC program provides another supporting case study

- Established in 1972, as a 2-year pilot program, the WIC program provides federal funds to states for supplemental foods, health care referrals, and nutrition education for low-income pregnant, breastfeeding, and non-breastfeeding postpartum women, as well as to infants and children up to age 5 who are found to be at nutritional risk

- The program became permanent in 1975 and over the years, evolved to provide very specific guidelines for food purchases, including
  - Monthly quantity guidelines designated by age
  - Ingredients (e.g., whole wheat vs. white grain)
  - Brand names

Note: WIC= Woman, Infants, and Children
Source: Oliveira et al. 2002. "The WIC program: background, trends, and issues." *United States Department of Agriculture: Economic Research Service.* Food Assistance and Nutrition Research Report No. 27.

Allowable WIC supplemental foods

- Juice
- WIC Formula
- Milk
- Breakfast cereal
- Cheese
- Eggs
- Whole wheat or whole grain bread
- Fish (canned)
- Legumes (dry) and/or peanut butter

- Beans, peas, lentils
- Brown rice
- Vegetables
- Fruits
- Soy beverage
- Tofu
- Yogurt
- Plain, dry, boxed infant cereal
- Baby food fruits/veggies/meats

Source: USDA: Food and Nutrition Service. "Women, infants and children (WIC): links to state agency WIC approved food." http://www.fns.usda.gov/wic/links-state-agency-wic-approved-food-lists (accessed January 5, 2015).

A recent change in guidelines seems to have had a positive impact on obesity rates among WIC children

- In 2009, the WIC program increased the value of vouchers provided to program participants toward the purchase of fruits and vegetables from $8 to $10[1]
- According to a report by the USDA (2012), obesity rates among children on WIC declined between 2008 and 2012[2]
    - Among children 1 year old:
        - 2008: 16.8% overweight
        - 2012: 15.3% overweight
    - Among children 2-4 years old:
        - 2008: 14.7% overweight
        - 2012: 14.0% overweight

Source: 1. *Federal Register*. 7 CFR Part 246, 2014, vol. 79 no. 54; 2. Johnson et al. 2013. "WIC Participant and Program Characteristics 2012." Prepared by Insight Policy Research under Contract No.AG-3198-C-11-0010. Alexandria, VA: U.S. Department of Agriculture, Food and Nutrition Service.

Make the healthy choice, the default choice by employing "nudging" techniques

Implement comprehensive strategies to increase adherence to healthier behaviors through
- Environmental nudges
- Economic nudges
- Educational nudges

Leverage opinion leaders and/ or influential settings to promote health through education programs

- "The American College of Sports Medicine (ACSM) recently completed a survey reporting that more than 80% of patients would pursue exercise if their physician advised them to do so.... A strong clear message from a trusted authority, such as the individual's personal physician, is a powerful motivator to adopt a more physically active lifestyle." [1]
- **Exercise is Medicine™** utilizes the highly regarded respect given to physicians as a leverage point to address unhealthy behaviors[2]
- **The Healthy Learner Model** connects health professionals with children in schools to provide education on how to manage their chronic diseases[3]

Source: 1) Phillips, E. 2008. "Exercise is Medicine: partnering with physicians." *ACSM's Health and Fitness Journal,* 13(6): 28-30; 2. Exercise is Medicine. "United States." http://www.exerciseismedicine.org/ (accessed November 4, 2014); 3. Warren-Boulton, E. 2013. "Redesigning the health care team: diabetes prevention and lifelong management." *National Institute of Health,* (13-7739):7-8.

Exercise is Medicine™ integrates discussion around the importance of behavioral choices within the healthcare setting

In 2010, Kaiser Permanente's Center for Health Research reviewed 13,562 abstracts and 474 articles to assist the Agency for Healthcare Research and Quality (AHRQ) update its recommendations on patient counselling by Primary Care Physicians to improve physical activity and diet. They found, that when counselled by a physician, participants in various studies....

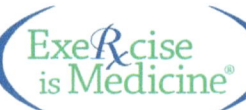

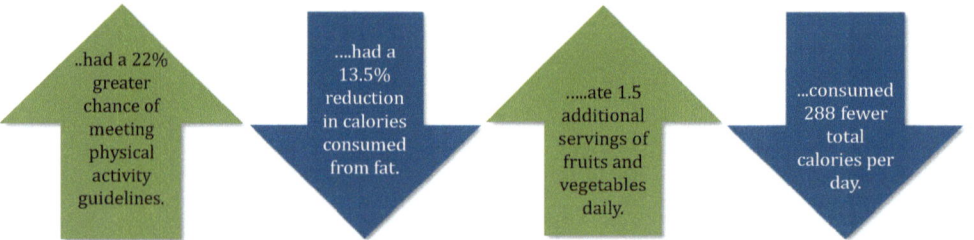

..had a 22% greater chance of meeting physical activity guidelines.

....had a 13.5% reduction in calories consumed from fat.

.....ate 1.5 additional servings of fruits and vegetables daily.

...consumed 288 fewer total calories per day.

Source: Phillips, E. 2008. "Exercise is Medicine: partnering with physicians." *ACSM's Health and Fitness Journal*, 13(6): 28-30.

91

The Healthy Learner model is designed to target students from kindergarten through grade 12

- Other than time spent sleeping, students spend more time in school than any other single activity[1]
- With the goal of maintaining students' health, the health learner model utilizes time spent in schools to coordinate care intervention programs to help students understand why their behavior choices impact their health[2]
- This model coordinates care through a team of professionals including
  - Health care professionals
  - School nurses specializing in chronic disease management
  - Students with chronic diseases and their families
  - School personnel
- This model is currently being used in Minneapolis Public Schools and St. Paul Public Schools to improve health of children with asthma

Source: 1. Bureau of Labor Statistics. 2014. "American time U.S. survey." http://www.bls.gov/tus/charts/ (accessed December 3, 2014); 2. Warren-Boulton, E. 2013. "Redesigning the health care team: diabetes prevention and lifelong management." *National Institute of Health*, (13-7739).

92

Outline

Physical activity can compensate for other poor health behaviors

Relative risk of mortality in relation to physical activity levels among those who currently smoke or are overweight/obese, 1986–1994

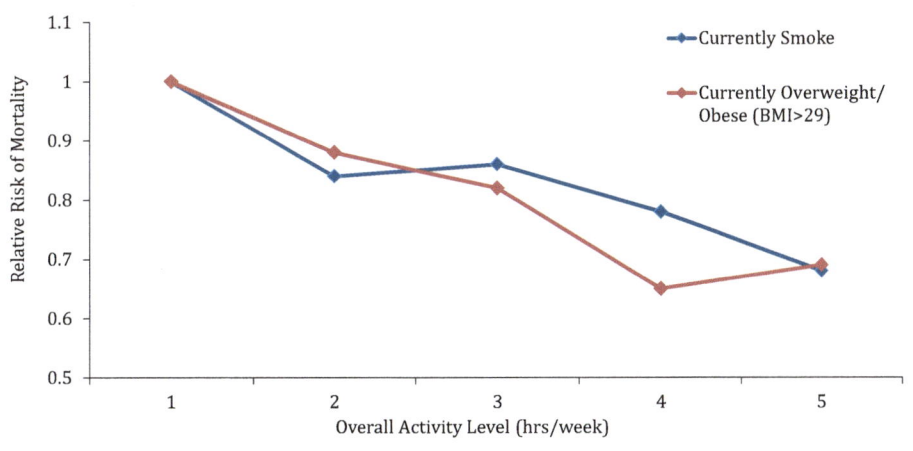

Source: Manson, J. 1999. "A prospective study of walking as compared with vigorous exercise in the prevention of coronary heart disease in women." *The New England Journal of Medicine*, 341:650-658.

In fact, physical activity "absolves many sins"

- Epidemiologic evidence suggests that just 30 min of daily moderate PA can result in substantial health benefits, including[1]
  - Lower risk of coronary heart disease and heart attacks
  - Lower risk of diabetes, various types of cancer and osteoporosis
  - Reduced pain associated with arthritis
  - Delayed onset of Alzheimer's and dementia
  - Longer life expectancy
- In fact, recent studies suggest that compared with 30 min of regular PA, prolonged bouts of strenuous PA do not necessarily multiply health and well-being[2]

Source: 1. Pratt, M. 1999. "Benefits of lifestyle activity vs structured exercise". *JAMA*, 281(4):375-376; 2. O'Keefe et al. 2014. "Exercising for heath and longevity vs peak performance: different regimens for different goals." *Mayo Clinic proceedings*. 89(9):171-1175.

ScienceDaily®
Your source for the latest research news

"Lack of exercise responsible for twice as many early deaths as obesity."

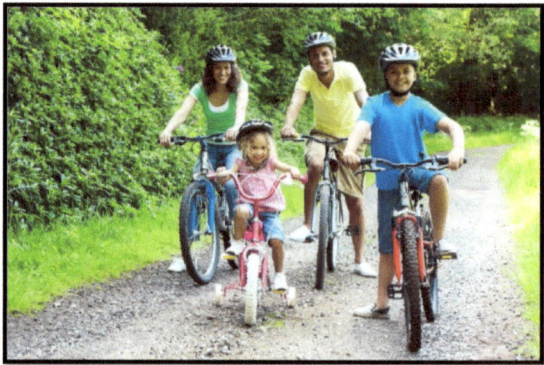

Source: University of Cambridge. "Lack of exercise responsible for twice as many early deaths as obesity." ScienceDaily. www.sciencedaily.com/releases/2015/01/150114143118.htm (accessed January 15, 2015); Photo credit: The Right Will/flikr.

Get at least 30 minutes of physical activity per day and the results could add years to your life

Physical Activity and Longevity in ~650,000 Adults

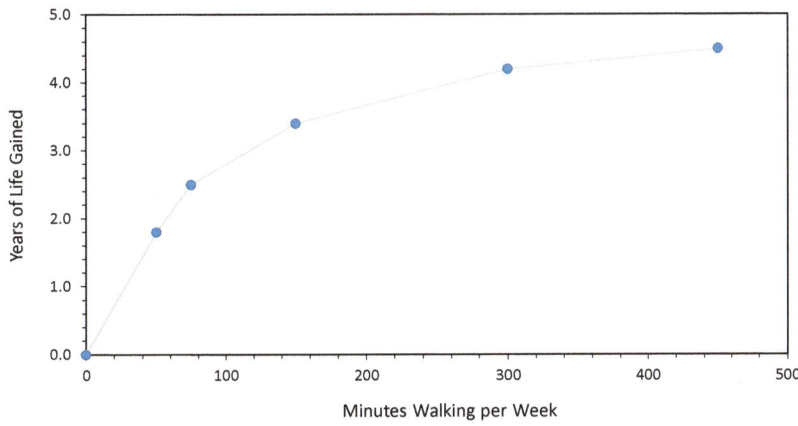

Source: Moore et al. 2012. "Leisure time physical activity of moderate to vigorous intensity and mortality: a large pooled cohort analysis. *PLoS Medicine.* 9(11): e1001335.

Physical activity is key

"...public health interventions that encourage people to make small but achievable changes in physical activity can have significant health benefits and may be easier to achieve and maintain (than efforts to reduce obesity)."

> -Dr. Nick Wareham, Director of the Medical Research Council, University of Cambridge

Source: University of Cambridge. "Lack of exercise responsible for twice as many early deaths as obesity." ScienceDaily. www.sciencedaily.com/releases/2015/01/150114143118.htm (accessed January 15, 2015).

Thus, we propose to focus on nudges that promote physical activity

1. Health benefit design
2. Exercise in schools
3. Work environments that encourage people to easily engage in walking 15-30 minutes/day

Specific recommendations for payers/ employers on health benefit design

- Eliminate co-pays and co-insurance for visits to coordinating, primary provider; evidence from Exercise is Medicine™ campaign suggests that providers can significantly influence patient behavior
- Vary premiums/deductibles on such factors as physical activity, tobacco use, weight, blood pressure, participation in workplace wellness programs
- Create other incentives that promote physical activity: where varying premiums and deductibles may not be an option, create financial incentives that promote physical activity

Example of other incentives for physical activity:

- Dr. Heather Royer, UC Santa Barbara working with a Fortune 500 company:
  - For four weeks company paid employees $10 per visit to gym for physical activity
  - After four weeks, employees offered a "commitment contract" where employee set money aside that they only received if they worked out over the next two months
  - Result after 3 years: 20% more of those with commitment contract still on regular physical activity

Source: Barro, J. "How to make yourself go to the gym." *The Upshot: Everyday Economics, The New York Times.* January 10, 2015.

Example of other incentives for physical activity

- The Alliance for a Healthier Minnesota in collaboration with RedBrick Health demonstrated the power of utilizing social networks to promote physical activity
- Employees were invited "to participate in team-based weight loss, physical activity and nutrition challenges over three months."
- 10,000 employees from Blue Cross and Blue Shield of Minnesota, Cargill, General Mills, HealthPartners, Medtronic, Target and UnitedHealth Group partook in the Challenge—competing with teams within their office, while concurrently competing against the other companies
- The results?
  - 37,000 lbs. lost and 16.5 million minutes of activity logged

Source: Rofling, K. 2011. "Good health is contagious: power of social media spreads healthy lifestyle." *CDCH Solutions,* January/February: 35-37.

Example of other incentives for physical activity:

- The "Anti-Charity Approach"[1]:
  - Set up an employee account with money from employer or employee or both
  - Establish a 'commitment contract' stating that if stipulated physical activity targets are not met, the funds in the account will go to an identified cause that the individual hates
  - Remember: Negative incentives often work better than positive ones[2]

Source: 1. Barro, J. "How to make yourself go to the gym." *The Upshot: Everyday Economics, The New York Times.* January 10, 2015; 2. Goldsmith, Kelly and Ravi Dhar. "To motivate, better to take away than to give." http://insight.kellogg.northwestern.edu/article/to_motivate_better_to_take_away_than_to_give/ (accessed January 15, 2015).

Example of other incentives for physical activity

- Be innovative
- Create a unique incentive that works for your work place and your work force

Thus, we propose to focus on nudges that promote physical activity

1. Health benefit design
2. Exercise in schools
3. Work environments that encourage people to easily engage in walking 15-30 minutes/day

Re-introduce exercise in schools

- Currently, less than 10% of schools provide daily physical education (PE) to students
- Significant time has been cut from PE and recess to increase time spent on academic subjects like reading and mathematics since the introduction of No Child Left Behind in 2001
- This is highly unfortunate given that
  - "Children who are more active show greater attention, have faster cognitive processing speed, and perform better on standardized academic tests than children who are less active."
  - "Physically active students are likely to be healthy and mentally sharp—attributes critical to being truly 'present' during the school day."

Source: Del Valle Cook et al. 2013. "Educating the student body: taking physical activity and physical education to school." *Institute of Medicine Report Brief.*

Re-introduce exercise in schools

- An Institute of Medicine committee recently recommended
  - An average of 30 minutes per day of physical education classes for elementary school students and an average of 45 minutes per day for middle and high school students
  - Additional physical activity, that should be incorporated throughout the school day, e.g., through recess and active classroom time
- The committee also felt that physical education should be designated as a core school subject; this may have the added benefit of students bringing these lessons home and thus positive spill-over effects to their parents/ families

Source: Del Valle Cook et al. 2013. "Educating the student body: taking physical activity and physical education to school." *Institute of Medicine Report Brief.*

Thus, we propose to focus on nudges that promote physical activity

1. Health benefit design
2. Exercise in schools
3. Work environments that encourage people to easily engage in walking 15-30 minutes/day

Design work spaces that promote physical activity

- The majority of U.S. adults spend a significant and increasing portion of their day at work
- Unfortunately, opportunities for physical activity in the workplace have declined significantly as a result of numerous technological advances that improve efficiency and productivity
- Given that physical inactivity is highly correlated with a variety of physical ailments, it is imperative to find ways to promote physical activity in the workplace
- A number of interventions can be incorporated into the workplace to promote physical activity, e.g., standing workstations, stepping devices, encouraging the use of stairs, etc.

Source: Carnethon et al. 2009. "Worksite wellness programs for cardiovascular disease prevention: a policy statement from the American Heart Association." *Circulation*, 120:1725-1741.

Design work spaces that promote physical activity

- Example interventions that can be incorporated into the workplace to promote physical activity:
  - Standing work spaces
  - Treadmill work stations
  - Policies of no elevator use if less than 4 flights
  - Parking spaces at least 15 minute walk to work area
  - Stand and stretch built into all meeting agendas
  - Walking meetings
  - Walking breaks

Design work spaces that promote physical activity

The Kaiser Permanente "Walking for workforce health toolkit" provides a comprehensive guide to promoting physical activity opportunities in the workplace:
http://www.slideshare.net/KaiserPermanente/kaiser-permanente-walking-for-workforce-health-toolkit

Many wise people have espoused physical activity for many years

"Lack of activity destroys the good condition of every human being, while movement and physical exercise save it and preserve it."

- Plato, (c. 428-347 B.C.)

Many wise people have espoused physical activity for many years

"Those who think they have not the time for bodily exercise will sooner or later have to find time for illness."

- Edward Stanley, 14th Early of Derby, British Statesman, 1873

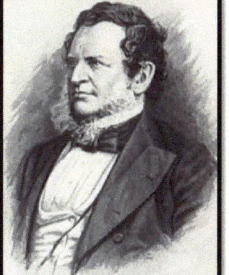

Photo credit: University of Nottingham, Manuscripts and Special Collections.
http://www.nottingham.ac.uk/manuscriptsandspecialcollections/learning/biographies/edwardgeorgegeoffreysmithstanley,14thearlofderby(1799-1869).aspx

113

Many wise people have espoused physical activity for many years

"Physical fitness is not only one of the most important keys to a healthy body, it is the basis of dynamic and creative intellectual activity."

- President John F. Kennedy, 1961

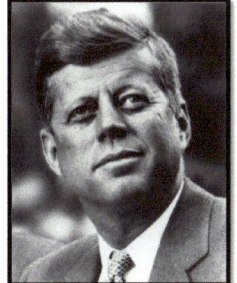

Photo credit: White House Press Office (WHPO).
http://www.jfklibrary.org/Page%20Not%20Found?item=%2fasset%2btree%2fasset%2bviewers%2fimage%2basset%2bviewer&user=extranet%5cAnonymous&site=website

114

But perhaps Idaho farm boy, Jim Rohn says it best…

"Take care of your body. It's the only place you have to live in."

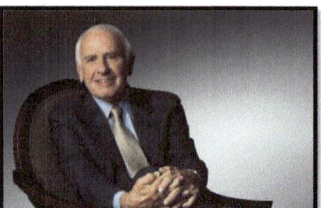

- James "Jim" Rohn, American entrepreneur, author and motivational speaker

---

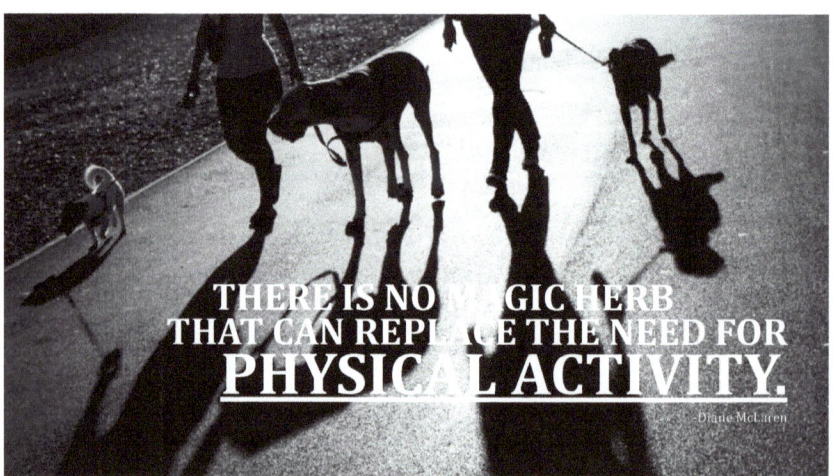

Photo Credit: Rborello/flickr.

www.ingramcontent.com/pod-product-compliance
Lightning Source LLC
Chambersburg PA
CBHW050751180526
45159CB00003B/1423